The School Of Sex: 20 Secrets On How To Improve In The Sack

Disclaimer and Terms of Use: Effort has been made to ensure that the information in this book is accurate and complete, however, the author and the publisher do not warrant the accuracy of the information, text and graphics contained within the book due to the rapidly changing nature of science, research, known and unknown facts and internet. The Author and the publisher do not hold any responsibility for errors, omissions or contrary interpretation of the subject matter herein. This book is presented solely for motivational and informational purposes only.

Table of Contents

Introduction

There are many men and women who suffer from low sex drive. Having a low sex drive can affect their relationship with the partner and it will cause low self esteem in some people with a low sex drive problem. Studies have shown that one in five men suffer from low libido. There are many factors which affect the sexual drive in men. Most of the men are in search of methods to improve in the sack. The sex drive in each person varies and there are various methods available to improve the sex drive and to increase the stamina of a person during the sexual act. Having sex offers many health benefits such as improved immune system, lowering blood pressure, lowering the risk of heart attacks, reducing the chances of prostate cancer, providing better sleep and reduces the stress levels. The important causes of low sexual drive and the various tips to overcome the problem are given below.

Psychological Problems

The sexual desire of a person gets affected by psychological issues. Problems in family life or problems in other relationship can cause stress during sexual performance. The strain and stress of daily life and anxiety caused by different reasons can also affect the libido of a person. Depression and other mental tensions can also have an adverse effect on the sexual desire and performance.

Medical Problems

Various health conditions such as obesity, high blood pressure, diabetes, heart problems. High cholesterol level and the medicines used for the treatment of various health issues can suppress the sexual desire. Drugs used for treating mental disorders, stress and HIV can also cause low sexual desire.

Changes In Hormone Levels

This is a major factor affecting the sexual performance in man as well as women. The level of the male sex hormone, testosterone is responsible for the sexual desire in man. The lower level of this hormone in men causes reduced sexual desire. The level of this hormone decreases with age, due to chronic diseases and due to the use of certain medications.

Lower Levels Of Dopamine

Sexual desire arises from the brain and the chemicals in the brain called dopamine are involved in transmitting the feeling. Lower levels of dopamine are seen in people with Parkinson's disease.

So, in order to improve the sexual desire the body should be healthy, devoid of tensions and stress and should have the perfect hormone levels. This can be achieved by proper diet, exercise and by practicing yoga and meditation. There are fruits and vegetables and other food items such as chocolates which function as an aphrodisiac and improve the sexual desire in man. The person should understand the situation and should make some effort to improve the condition. One can try different simple tips to increase the sexual desire if there are no particular health problems causing the low sexual desire. Better bonding between the partners and introducing new methods in sex life can improve the sexual desire to a certain extent. Concentrating on the pleasure experienced from the act of sex rather than concentrating on the physical performance will give better confidence and will increase the sexual drive. Solving any of the conflicts with your partner can also help in improving the sexual desire.

20 Tips To Improve Your Sex Life

It is really difficult to find a person who is not interested to improve on his or her sex life. Everyone feels that they need to learn more about sex all the time to make their partner that much happier in the sack. The following are some of the tips that you can try out to improve your sex life and to floor your partner whenever you have sex.

Make Yourself Look Attractive

Men are attracted to women who wear attractive looking clothes. It has been researched and found out that men are really interested in women wearing crimson color. Men feel that women look really attractive in hue of red and also love their women to spend a lot of time on a date in red.

- Men love to have sex with women who look stunning in red color dresses.
- They develop sexual urge and drive whenever they get close and personal to women in red.
- Men will also perform better in bed with a woman in red and hence it is better for you to also think of wearing red lingerie whenever you want to have passionate sex.

Chart Out An Exercise Routine

It is important for you to be really fit, active and healthy to be a good sex performer. There is no room for lethargy during sex as this would really put off your partner. It is important for you to schedule an exercise routine at least five times a week to make you more flexible and also give you a boost of power that you will need whenever you get to bed with your partner. The following are some of the exercises that you need to work on to improve your sex life:

- Flexibility is very essential component for sex and yoga is the best way to make your body flexible. Try yoga and other stretching exercises to enhance your flexibility in bed.

- There are many different types of positions that you can try out during a sexual intercourse. This will bring in a lot of passion to your sex life. But, you need to have strong muscles to perform some of the amazing sexual intercourse positions. Strength training and endurance workouts will help you to tone your muscles to be a better performer in bed.

- Cardio exercises are very important for you to be a good performer on the sack. It will keep your heart strong and will also help in charging your body. You can try out swimming, jogging, walking or running about 25 to 30 minutes at least four days a week to perform better during sex.

Take A Proper Diet

The amount of calories that you intake will have a telling effect on the stamina and your performance in bed. You will only be having the perfect stamina and the strength to be a better sex performer if you stick to a healthy diet.

- Eating a lot of fresh fruits and vegetables will help in providing the necessary minerals, vitamins, and fiber that is needed for the body.

- Vegetables will provide you with high levels of energy as well as takes care of your muscle tissues to keep you strong.

- They will also help in removing the stress levels from your body so that you are very good when it comes to sex.

Talk Before And During Sex

Communication is a key element that will lead to happy and enjoyable sessions in bed. It is vital that you communicate with your partner not just before the sex, but also while having sex.

- You need to be very open to your partner and tell what sex position that you like, what your sexual fantasies are and what you are expecting from your partner.

- You will find that sex is more fun and pleasurable when you open up your mind to your partner.

- Silence will take you nowhere during sex and being accommodative and frank through an open channel of communication will throw away all the sexual problems out of the window.

New Sex Positions

You need to be adventurous in bed and this might even entice your partner to be more active during your love making sessions.

- It is important for you to try new sex positions every time you hit the bed with your partner.

- You need to talk about the new sex position that you are going to try out to take your partner in your stride so that you do not face any rejections during sex.

- You will not gain any depth by forcing your partner to try out a new sex position. The passion for new sex positions should come from both sides to make it enjoyable and pleasurable.

Foreplay Is Very Important

There will be no passion or attraction when you try to push your partner in bed to have a quick intercourse session. Neither you nor your partner would be able to enjoy sex this way. Foreplay is a very important sex act that you should try out to provide the best sexual experience for both you and your partner.

- Concentrating on foreplay before the big bang will make your partner more responsive your thrusts and pushes and you will experience the best sex that you have ever had in your life.

- You can even try out certain sexual messages in the middle of the day or even have a little bit of phone sex with your partner in the middle of the day that will help in improving the passion while having sex at night.

- Physical foreplay techniques like kissing your partner from head to toe, sucking his or her nipples, a little bit of oral sex and so on is sure to ignite passion in your partner which will lead to a pleasurable intercourse session.

Concentrate On Physical Affection

If you feel that your partner is not aroused by your actions in bed despite you performing better in bed, then you need to try to woo your partner and develop a physical bonding with your partner.

- Kissing, cuddling and embracing your partner whenever he or she is in distress or upset about some problem or the other will help you to maintain an emotional bond with your partner.

- You can give your partner passionate kisses as well as fondle their private parts ever so gently in a bid to maintain your physical bond and this could result in having a steamy session in bed.

Keep Your Partner Informed About Changes In Your Body

- It is very important for you to spill out all the problems that you are facing to your partner so that he or she is not kept in the dark when having an intercourse.

- You might be feeling hot flashes at night or your vagina might be getting dry due to menopause. You need to be open about these things with your partner so that he knows the exact situation and can adjust accordingly.

- If you are no longer excited about the thought of having sex and do not get an erection when you talk about sex, then you need to inform your partner about the same so that she can try to stimulate you in different ways to bring your manhood to life.

Quit Smoking And Reduce Alcohol Intake

- Smoking will affect the flow of blood to the penis, vaginal tissues and clitoris and thereby you will lack the sexual desire and drive to be a good performer in bed.

- Women who smoke also tend to attain menopause earlier than non smokers and men feel their manhood does not have the energy and stamina to perform in bed. Hence, quitting smoking will help both men and women to enjoy sex better and for a long time.

- Having one drink a day will help you to be a good performer in bed as you will be able to relax better.

- But, if you are a heavy drinker, then you will be suffering from erectile dysfunction as a man and women will suffer from hot flashes and disrupted sleep.

Give Time For Sex As You Age

You will not be at your sexual best in your 40s and would be a poorer performer than what you had achieved when you were in your late 20s. There is no doubt that your sexual responses will be slower as you age.

- It is important for you to understand that both you and your partner will need more time to get sexually aroused as well as to reach orgasm as you age.

- It is not a bad idea to spend more time to have sex and to reach the climax and never be frustrated that you are not climaxing very soon.

- You can think of a little bit of oral sex to arouse your partner for sex.

Lesson Sex Session

One of the best ways to offer better sex to your partner is to consider a lesson session on sex.

- Get suggestions from both partners on what type of sex position and sexual fantasy that they would like and one that they have not yet tried out.

- All you need to do is to choose the better suggestion between the two and get down in bed instantly.

- Most of the time you would be thinking that you know what your partner wants when it comes to sex and by offering a chance for an open suggestion you get better sex suggestions from your partner which can take you to the height of intimacy.

Massage

One of the ways to drive your partner into a steamy hot sex session with you is to give him or her a nice massage. A sensual touch by the fingers of your partner or even by his or her smooth body over your body is sure to power up the sexual energy flow in you and you will be able to perform better in bed.

- You can unlock your partner's body with a relaxing and sensual massage and could drive you and your partner to experience intense orgasms.

- You will also be able to relax your partner and to give him or her the best sensual touches that will make them to be a better performer in bed.

- A sensual oral sex at the end of the sensual massage will drive your partner to get on top of you and to perform sex like never before.

Play Games In Bed

- Playing a pack of cards or a strip poker game is the best way for better sex. You can add intense passion to your love life by offering a chance to the winner to choose any sex action that they want the loser to perform on their body.

- You should limit this action for a minute or two and this game of seduction will drive you both to finally end up enjoying steamy sex session.

- The great thing about such games is that you get a chance to ask the other person to do things that they have not yet done and will help in better sex.

Dirty Talk

Many people get turned on when they hear dirty talk. It is one of the easiest ways to indulge a person into sex and you find them respond to sexual words easily and without any hitch.

- Uttering some of the most pleasant sex talk that your partner loves to hear will drive then emotionally and sensually that they will get aroused and will be ready to have a good sex session with you.

- You need to be very careful with this art of talking dirty and it must not be done badly in a manner that it would result in just getting a few giggles from your partner rather than driving them to sex craving.

- You can talk about how you feel being inside her, how much you enjoy getting horny with your partner and so on that will help in enjoying better sex.

- You need to practice dirty talking a bit before exploding it on your partner for the first time. You must only talk about positive words and never include insult words in your dirty talk.

Try New Places For Sex

It could be boring to have sex in the same place every time. You need to change the place where you have sex sometimes like how you change your intercourse positions for better enjoyment.

- Shifting to a new place to have sex will ignite the passion of both the partners to a higher level of ecstasy and excitement.

- You can think of parking your car in a dark and secluded place and indulge in sex. You are sure to enjoy it to the fullest.

- Another option that you can try out, if you are bold enough, is a public place that is not too public.

- You can even think of having sex in your kitchen or your dining table or your balcony or even in someone else's home. By trying out different places for having sex you will be increasing your pleasure and your drive to have sex.

Use Of Sex Toys

Another option to excite your partner and to enjoy pleasurable sex is to use sex toys as a tool for foreplay. You can think of cock rings for male partners and dildos for female partners. Titillating your partner's sex organs with sex toys will arouse them in such a manner that they will offer you better sex sessions that result in intense orgasms. Sex toys can be used to arouse your partner and to get him or her on the offensive in bed.

Tease Your Partner Into Sex

If you and your partner have been having sex for a long time and sex happens automatically for you, then there is every chance that you have lost the passion and vigor that is associated with sexual intercourse. You can bring back the intensity and passion into your sex life by implementing a few changes in your sex life.

- You need to start to enjoy the sensuality of sex and never concentrate on the end part of the sex.

- You should try to tease your partner to lay you on the bed and this can be done by getting undressed in front of him or her or wearing sexy and revealing clothes.

- If you are carrying out the art of sensual touching, then you need to make sure that you communicate your love and sexual passion to your partner through your touch.

- If you are the receiver, then you need to moan and express the feelings that you are enjoying for each end every stroke of your partner. This will ignite your partner to perform even better sensually and you both will end up enjoying a very good climax.

Helping Partner In Household Chores

Sharing the duties of childcare and household chores between two partners can bring about a beautiful and healthy sexual relationship between the two. Helping your partner out in day to day household chores will drive them to be more than satisfied being in relationship with you and will drive them to have more sex with you. In fact, it has been found out that doing daily chores is a kind of foreplay that will drive your homemaker to be a wily old fox in bed and provide you with ultimate sex pleasure that you have never experienced. Thanking your partner with a kiss or a soft cuddle or even exciting his or her private parts for helping you out in daily chores will make him or her good performer in bed.

Talking At The Right Time

It is very important for you to open your mind and let out all your sexual conversations to excite your partner and to make him or her perform even better during sex.

- There are two different types of sexual conversations that people have normally: one is when they are having sex and the other is talking about sex elsewhere.

- It is really important for you to express your love, pleasure and the way you feel when your partner is caressing you and playing with your private parts. You need to tell these things out immediately to excite your partner so that he or she explores your body even better.

- You need to wait to get to a neutral setting whenever you want to express your larger problems like: orgasm troubles or lack of sexual desire. If you express this in the middle of a sex session, there is every chance that this might turn your partner off and he or she will also lose the sexual drive forever.

You should never be performing sex just to please your partner or to protect your partner's feelings. The sex drive must come from the inside and this is the only way you and your partner will be able to enjoy a sex session.

- It is important for you to open your mind to your partner if you are facing any sexual problems.

- Faking an orgasm or giving false smiles can put your partner off and he or she will also not be able to offer you good sex sessions.

- Every sexual problem can be solved if both partners can talk it across as this conversation will also lead them to finding a clue to solve the sexual problem that they are facing.